DECIPHERING DEMENTIA

Understanding and Treating Cognitive Decline in Dementia

Dr. Harmony Wells

Copyright © by Dr. Harmony wells 2024. All rights reserved.

Before this document is Duplicated or reproduced in any manner, the publisher's consent must be gained. Therefore, the contents within can neither be stored electronically, transferred, nor kept in a database. Neither in Part nor in full can the document be copied, scanned, faxed, or retained without approval from the publisher or creator.

TABLE OF CONTENT

INTRODUCTION

Investigating cognitive decline in depth provides an opportunity to learn about the complex processes of the human mind and the difficulties people encounter in understanding this phenomenon. In the talk that follows, we will explore the various facets of cognitive decline, looking at its basic principles, causes, and early warning signs, in an effort to provide readers a thorough grasp of this widespread problem.

The phrase "cognitive decline" refers to a range of cognitive impairments, from milder issues with memory and attention to more serious ailments like dementia. Fundamentally, cognitive decline is the progressive loss of cognitive abilities such as attention, language, memory, and problem-solving. Investigating the fundamental causes of these alterations is necessary to comprehend this idea.

There is a wide range of factors that can influence the causes of cognitive decline, including age, genetics, lifestyle, and underlying medical disorders. Even while aging naturally causes changes in cognition, it's important to recognize the difference between pathological cognitive decline brought on by diseases like Alzheimer's disease or other types of dementia and normal age-related decline.

We disentangle the complexities of cognitive decline in this first chapter by looking at the complicated interactions between biological, psychological, and environmental factors. Investigating how hereditary features can predispose people to particular cognitive problems highlights the influence of genetics on cognitive health. Furthermore, a person's lifestyle decisions, career, and level of schooling all have a significant impact on how resilient or vulnerable their cognitive abilities are.

Early symptoms and signs are important markers for identifying cognitive deterioration. The fact that memory loss, concentration issues, and difficulties solving problems might appear subtly emphasizes the significance of early detection. This chapter clarifies these early indicators and highlights the need of taking preventative action to address cognitive problems before they become more severe.

In order to provide a conclusive understanding of the fundamental causes of cognitive loss, diagnostic approaches to dementia are essential. We explore the range of techniques used by medical practitioners, such as laboratory testing, brain imaging, and cognitive evaluations. Through the process of deconstructing the diagnostic process, readers are able to comprehend how medical professionals deal with the difficulties involved in recognizing and classifying cognitive diseases.

Understanding the various forms of cognitive decline requires an understanding of dementia kinds. Within the larger spectrum of cognitive illnesses, Alzheimer's disease, vascular dementia, Lewy body dementia, and frontotemporal dementia are separate entities. This chapter provides guidance by explaining the traits and particular difficulties connected to each kind of dementia.

Cognitive decline treatment is a multimodal approach that addresses disease modification as well as symptomatic alleviation. In order to manage cognitive symptoms, medications, cognitive treatment, and lifestyle modifications are essential. Through the examination of these tactics, readers acquire a thorough comprehension of the instruments at their disposal in the endeavor to alleviate the consequences of cognitive aging.

Dementia prevention and lifestyle interventions emphasize the proactive steps people can take to support cognitive health. This chapter highlights the impact of lifestyle choices in potentially avoiding or postponing cognitive decline, from promoting social relationships and stimulating cognitive activities to keeping a healthy diet and getting regular exercise.

Providing assistance to both persons and carers is a vital part of managing cognitive decline. The effects on people and their families are significant, and this chapter addresses the difficulties caretakers encounter while offering suggestions for creating a nurturing atmosphere. There is a thorough discussion of methods for preserving quality of life and improving the wellbeing of those who are experiencing cognitive impairment as well as their carers.

The pursuit of efficacious therapies and treatments is aided by the promising developments in dementia research. This chapter gives readers an overview of the rapidly changing field of dementia research by exploring the most recent scientific findings, which range from novel therapy methods to biomarker studies.

Targeted therapies to improve daily living skills and cognitive performance are provided by cognitive rehabilitation strategies. Those with cognitive decline can make significant progress in some domains of functioning with tailored exercises and techniques. This chapter provides insights into the possible advantages of cognitive rehabilitation by examining its guiding principles and practical implementations.

Future directions for cognitive health interventions are illuminated by promising treatments that are approaching. This chapter offers an overview of the cutting-edge strategies that could advance dementia therapy in the years to come, from experimental medications that target particular pathways to cutting-edge technology like virtual reality.

The preservation of an individual's autonomy, dignity, and quality of life is crucial when it comes to dementia care, and this is especially true when ethical considerations come into play. This chapter examines the moral conundrums that challenge caregivers, families, and healthcare professionals. It offers advice on how to make difficult choices while maintaining the values of respect and decency.

Testimonials from individuals who have overcome cognitive decline provide motivation and fortitude in the face of difficulty. Readers are given a fuller insight of the human experience and the resilience that may be shown in the face of cognitive decline by reading the accounts of people who have successfully navigated the difficulties posed by cognitive illnesses.

Resources for further support offer a thorough guide for anyone looking for community resources, help, and extra information about cognitive decline. For individuals seeking to comprehend and manage cognitive problems, this chapter provides a helpful road map that they can use to contact online support groups, helplines, or educational resources.

To sum up, this investigation into understanding dementia has tried to give readers a comprehensive grasp of cognitive decline, from its theoretical underpinnings to useful approaches for mitigating its effects. We hope to add to the body of information that will enable patients, caregivers, and medical professionals to make better decisions regarding their cognitive health by deciphering the complexity of cognitive decline.

CHAPTER ONE

Unveiling the Complexity of Dementia

We are invited to travel through the many facets, difficulties, and facets of dementia, a profound and complex disease that affects cognitive abilities. The investigation "Unveiling the Complexity of Dementia" takes readers through the genetic influences, environmental factors, neurobiological complexities, and lived experiences that together define the complex landscape of dementia in an effort to shed light on the condition's varied nature.

The understanding that a person's genetic makeup influences both their vulnerability and resilience to dementia lies at the heart of this investigation. One's susceptibility to particular types of cognitive decline is greatly influenced by their family history, which is entwined with hereditary characteristics. This chapter establishes the foundation for tailored interventions by revealing the genetic components at play and emphasizing the necessity of developing strategies that take the individual's distinct genetic composition into account.

The narrative surrounding cognitive health is complexly shaped by environmental influences.

Individuals' cognitive resilience is shaped by a confluence of factors including lifestyle decisions, educational attainment, and socioeconomic circumstances. In exploring the external elements that add to dementia's complexity, this chapter emphasizes the importance of modifiable risk factors. By revealing avenues for promoting cognitive well-being, an understanding of this interaction promotes the creation of interventions and preventive measures that take the larger environmental context into account.

Understanding the influence of dementia on cognitive functions centers on the complex neuronal landscape of the brain. Memory loss, poor judgment, and behavioral abnormalities are signs of disruptions in brain networks. Readers will have a greater understanding of the difficulties faced by dementia patients by learning about these intricate neurological details. A person's cognitive and emotional well-being are significantly impacted by the progressive nature of cognitive decline, which is not only a cognitive journey but also a complicated dance inside the intricate web of the brain's functioning.

The fact that dementia comes in many forms complicates matters further. Frontotemporal dementia, Lewy body dementia, vascular dementia, and Alzheimer's disease are different conditions with different traits. Examining these variations helps to identify the various ways that cognitive diseases present, leading to a more sophisticated approach to diagnosis and therapy. By revealing the distinct characteristics of every subtype, medical practitioners can customize interventions to tackle the particular difficulties encountered by individuals and their carers.

Early symptoms and signs are like little bells that gently announce the arrival of cognitive impairment. It becomes essential to recognize these subtleties in order to act promptly. This chapter explores the nuances of early detection and highlights the significance of being acutely aware of tiny changes that could be missed otherwise. By identifying chances for early interventions and assistance, the unraveling of these indicators sets the foundation for cooperative efforts to improve the trajectory of cognitive health.

A crucial component of comprehending the intricacy of dementia is the use of diagnostic techniques. Healthcare practitioners employ genetic testing, brain imaging, and cognitive evaluations to identify underlying causes. The diagnostic process is characterized by both obstacles and advances, necessitating a thorough and dynamic strategy. Through navigating the complexity of the diagnostic landscape, this investigation acknowledges how our understanding is constantly changing and how diagnostic tools are being improved.

The lived experiences of individuals with dementia and their carers weave the human dimension into the intricacy of the disease. Narratives from personal experience offer significant perspectives on the psychological, social, and pragmatic difficulties encountered by individuals experiencing cognitive decline. By revealing these stories, readers are welcomed into the personal battles and victories, encouraging compassion and empathy in tackling the complex issues related to dementia. These tales humanize dementia, highlighting the value of person-centered care and the necessity of an all-encompassing strategy to assist individuals who are impacted by the disease.

"Unveiling the Complexity of Dementia" concludes with providing an overview of the many facets of this illness. The story aims to foster a deep comprehension of dementia by interpreting hereditary, environmental, neurological, and experiential factors. A road to compassionate treatment, creative solutions, and a team effort to decipher the nuances of cognitive health are made clear by this insight. The route is not finished; it is characterized by a never-ending pursuit of knowledge, compassion, and a dedication to improving the lives of those impacted by this complex illness.

CHAPTER TWO

Understanding the Cognitive Landscape

The cognitive landscape is a vast and complex area that entices us to go on an intriguing voyage into the inner workings of the human mind. A tour guide through the many domains of cognition, "Understanding the Cognitive Landscape" provides information on language, attention, memory, problem-solving, and the neurological underpinnings that all influence our cognitive experience.

The fascinating domain of attention is central to the landscape of cognition. This cognitive filter selects from among the many inputs in our environment what warrants our attention. Comprehending attention reveals the selective mechanisms that impact perception, directing people to give priority to some information over others. The focus of this investigation is on attention's function as a conduit for cognitive interaction with the outside environment.

A fundamental component of cognitive functioning, memory is a complicated terrain that is divided into discrete regions for sensory, short-term, and long-term memory. The processes of encoding, storing, and retrieving information influence memory and recall in a complex way. The study of memory explores the processes that underlie learning and influence our capacity to pick up information and adjust to a constantly changing environment.

The expressive and rich domain of language adds complexity to the cognitive environment. This investigation reveals the various mechanisms that control how language influences cognition and communication, from the difficulties of language comprehension to speech production. The variety of languages and the significant influence of language skills on social interactions and cultural expression enhance the cognitive landscape.

Within the cognitive landscape, problem-solving appears as a dynamic terrain where people negotiate difficulties, reach decisions, and come up with plans to get over roadblocks. The goal of this chapter is to dissect the mental processes that go into solving problems, illuminating how the mind gathers data, comes up with answers, and adjusts to unfamiliar circumstances. The ability to solve problems is essential for navigating the difficulties of daily life and demonstrates the changing character of cognition.

Throughout life, the cognitive landscape changes; it is not a static tableau. Knowing the dynamic nature of cognitive functions enhances our understanding of the human mind, from infancy cognitive developments to aging-related changes. Cognitive shifts in later life highlight the significance of maintaining cognitive health and adjusting to age-related changes, while childhood cognitive milestones like language acquisition and spatial reasoning provide the groundwork for lifetime learning.

The foundation of the cognitive landscape is made up of neurobiological principles, with complex brain networks conducting the symphony of cognitive processes. The chapter explores the structure and function of the brain, revealing how different brain areas, neurotransmitters, and neurons shape the cognitive experience. Gaining insight into the neural underpinnings of cognition allows one to better appreciate the interaction between the intricate workings of the brain and its physical architecture. The brain's capacity for self-reorganization in response to experience, or neuroplasticity, highlights the dynamic character of the cognitive landscape and the possibility of adaptability and lifelong learning.

The importance of cognitive diversity becomes clear as we move through the cognitive landscape. The diverse range of cognitive abilities and difficulties among individuals adds to the intricate fabric of human cognition. This investigation highlights the significance of appreciating and honoring cognitive variety, encouraging a broad comprehension of the diverse ways that people traverse their cognitive environments. Cognitive diversity promotes group creativity and problem-solving through a range of learning styles and approaches to problem-solving.

To sum up, "Understanding the Cognitive Landscape" is a journey through the complex realm of human perception and thought. Through an exploration of the complexities surrounding attention, memory, language, problem-solving, and the neurological underpinnings of cognition, this chapter equips readers with the necessary tools to successfully navigate the cognitive terrain. Our collective perception of what it means to be human is shaped by the insights we acquire from a deeper knowledge of the cognitive processes that characterize the human experience. These insights go beyond individual cognition. A rich and dynamic tapestry, the cognitive landscape encourages further investigation and fosters a greater understanding of the intricacies that characterize our cognitive journey.

CHAPTER THREE

Early Signs and Symptoms of Cognitive Decline

Understanding the early warning signs and symptoms of cognitive decline is an important research endeavor with broad ramifications for patients, their families, and the medical community. The goal of this thorough analysis is to identify the subtle but significant indicators that indicate the beginning of cognitive changes, highlighting the significance of early diagnosis as a means of facilitating prompt intervention and assistance.

Delays in memory are frequently the first signs of cognitive deterioration. People frequently encounter momentary amnesia in their daily lives, such as misplacing keys or momentarily forgetting a name. But if these errors start to happen more frequently and affect regular duties and tasks, they might be a sign of underlying cognitive abnormalities. It is important to identify these memory lapses early on since it allows for a more thorough investigation of any possible cognitive changes and motivates people to get evaluated by a professional.

Other early indicators of cognitive deterioration include trouble focusing and staying focused. Things that you used to do with easy could become difficult, which would make you less productive and frustrated. Early identification of these attentional difficulties enables people to seek support and put coping mechanisms in place to lessen the effects on their everyday activities, relationships, and jobs. The person's capacity to manage cognitive changes can be greatly improved by using this proactive strategy.

Early cognitive decline might also present with language impairments. People could have trouble putting their ideas into words, following and contributing to conversations, or finding the appropriate phrases. Even though they are initially minor, these linguistic roadblocks highlight the complex relationship between language and cognitive function. Early detection of these linguistic alterations enables prompt support and intervention, addressing the cognitive factors affecting communication.

A major symptom of cognitive impairment is impaired judgment and decision-making. People could make bad financial judgments, find it difficult to make wise choices in different situations, or ignore safety issues. It becomes critical to recognize these early indicators for the person and those in their support system. It makes it possible to take preventative action to deal with possible outcomes, protecting one's financial and personal security.

Early indicators of cognitive deterioration may include alterations in spatial orientation and visual perception. Even though they may appear gradually, challenges with familiar space navigation, distance estimation, or visual information interpretation can have a significant impact on day-to-day functioning. When these spatial limitations are identified early on, people are more likely to seek evaluations and treatments that address possible underlying cognitive problems, which may lessen the impact on tasks requiring spatial awareness.

A deterioration in cognitive function may manifest as subtle but significant symptoms such as social disengagement and personality changes. People may demonstrate changes in their personality traits, become less interested in social contacts, or become more reserved. An in-depth examination of the emotional and social ramifications of cognitive decline is made possible by early recognition of these changes. In order to navigate the difficulties brought on by cognitive changes, it fosters understanding and empathy through open communication among support networks.

Individuals who are going through cognitive decline may find daily chores that used to feel ordinary to be more difficult. Early in the course of cognitive changes, challenges with budgeting, scheduling, and activity planning and organization may arise. Early detection of these difficulties enables the application of supporting measures to preserve autonomy and standard of living. It gives people the confidence to experiment with adaptable methods and take part in activities that enhance cognitive health.

Sensitivity and awareness are necessary when approaching the identification of early indicators and symptoms of cognitive deterioration. Although these signs might point to underlying cognitive problems, they can also be caused by a number of other things, such as stress, exhaustion, or illnesses. It is critical to get expert assessment and assistance in order to precisely determine the type and severity of cognitive abnormalities. Early intervention provides the chance to address risk factors that can be changed and to put methods into place that may delay the rate at which cognitive decline develops.

In summary, investigating the early warning signs and symptoms of cognitive decline is a complex process that necessitates a thorough comprehension. Understanding the complexities of memory loss, attention problems, language barriers, poor judgment, changes in spatial orientation, personality changes, and difficulties with daily chores helps us better understand the variety of ways that cognitive decline manifests itself. This knowledge emphasizes how crucial early detection is in serving as a spark for prompt assistance and response. Through cultivating consciousness, candid dialogue, and a dedication to cognitive health, we augment a group endeavor to confront cognitive aging with compassion, comprehension, and a commitment to improving the lives of individuals impacted.

CHAPTER FOUR

Diagnostic Approaches to Dementia

Dementia diagnosis is a multifaceted process that requires careful navigation of several roads through the difficult terrain of cognitive health. In the process of deciphering this illness, medical practitioners employ a wide range of diagnostic techniques, each of which adds a distinct dimension to the collective comprehension. The field of dementia diagnosis necessitates a multimodal strategy that changes with our understanding, incorporating everything from genetic testing to cognitive evaluations and brain imaging.

Cognitive evaluations: Providing a thorough analysis of a person's cognitive abilities, cognitive evaluations are the cornerstone of dementia diagnosis. These evaluations consist of a series of exams that investigate verbal, memory, attention, and problem-solving skills. Because these tests are standardized, it is easier to track changes in cognitive performance over time and to establish a baseline. The finer points identified by cognitive evaluations help distinguish between dementia subtypes, enabling medical practitioners to identify particular cognitive impairments suggestive of underlying neurodegenerative processes.

Brain Imaging Techniques: By providing a visual examination of the structural and functional changes inside the brain, brain imaging techniques broaden the diagnostic landscape. Computed Tomography (CT) and Magnetic Resonance Imaging (MRI) scans offer fine-grained pictures that show dementia-related lesions, atrophy, or structural abnormalities. On the other hand, metabolic activity is highlighted in Positron Emission Tomography (PET) scans, which display patterns that may point to particular subtypes of dementia. These imaging modalities improve the accuracy of characterizing the underlying brain pathology and play a major role in the diagnosis process.

Genetic Testing: When a familial connection is indicated, the genetic component adds another level of difficulty to the diagnosis of dementia. When it comes to determining certain gene changes linked to inherited types of dementia, including frontotemporal dementia or familial Alzheimer's disease, genetic testing becomes an invaluable tool. Knowing a person's genetic composition helps determine their prognosis and helps family members calculate their risk. Genetic testing is important when there is a suspicion of a hereditary component, even though it is not always used.

Cerebrospinal Fluid Analysis: This more intrusive yet informative method uses biochemical markers linked to dementia to analyze cerebrospinal fluid. In the cerebral fluid, elevated concentrations of tau and beta-amyloid proteins point to underlying neurodegenerative processes. Cerebrospinal fluid analysis is less frequently used than other diagnostic techniques, but it provides extra information to support the overall diagnosis, especially in research settings and specialized dementia clinics.

Neuropsychological Testing: Offering a thorough examination of cognitive, emotional, and behavioral functions, neuropsychological testing delves deeper into cognitive evaluation. These tests explore particular domains including language, visuospatial ability, and executive function, going beyond the scope of traditional cognitive examinations. A more thorough cognitive profile is produced by neuropsychological testing, which helps with the differential diagnosis of different forms of dementia. This method works especially well for capturing the subtleties of a person's cognitive advantages and disadvantages.

Clinical and Medical History: Compiling a thorough individual's clinical and medical history is a fundamental step in the diagnosis procedure. Investigating the beginning and development of symptoms, prior medical issues, prescription drugs, and family history are all part of this comprehensive approach. Healthcare providers can rule out other possible causes for symptoms, such as drug side effects or medical disorders that mirror dementia, by placing an individual's cognitive decline within the context of their whole medical and personal history.

Collaborative and Interdisciplinary Approach: The diagnostic process is distinguished by a collaborative and interdisciplinary approach, which acknowledges the multidimensional nature of dementia. Together, neurologists, geriatricians, neuropsychologists, and other medical specialists evaluate results, pool knowledge, and guarantee a thorough assessment. This cooperative endeavor recognizes that dementia is a complicated illness that calls for a range of viewpoints in order to improve diagnostic precision and deliver comprehensive care.

To sum up, the diagnostic methods for dementia comprise a variety of evaluations, imaging methods, genetic understandings, and teamwork. The intricate structure of cognitive health is reflected in the multiple routes that healthcare providers must negotiate. The environment of diagnosis changes in tandem with our growing understanding of dementia, providing hope for earlier and more accurate diagnoses. For dementia patients and their families, this new strategy offers the possibility of more individualized therapies and enhanced quality of life. The diagnostic process becomes a tool of elucidating the intricacies of dementia as well as a conduit for individualized assistance and care.

CHAPTER FIVE

Navigating the Types of Dementia

The state of dementia is intricate and multidimensional, encompassing a wide range of subtypes, each distinguished by unique characteristics and underlying illnesses. Understanding the several forms of dementia, its distinctive symptoms, diagnostic difficulties, and possible ramifications for patients and their families, is essential for navigating this complex terrain.

Disease of Alzheimer's:
With Alzheimer's disease accounting for the majority of dementia cases, it is the most common and well-known type of dementia. It is typified by the build-up of tau tangles and beta-amyloid plaques in the brain, which causes neurodegeneration to develop. Behavior changes, memory loss, and cognitive impairment are common symptoms of Alzheimer's disease. Managing Alzheimer's entails addressing the disease's slow progression, realizing how it affects day-to-day functioning, and investigating therapies to improve cognitive health.

Dementia Vascular:
Impaired blood flow to the brain, frequently as a result of strokes or other vascular problems, is the cause of vascular dementia. The progressive deterioration of cognitive abilities is the hallmark of this kind of dementia, and the symptoms differ based on the site of vascular injury. Managing cardiovascular health risk factors, treating the effects of strokes, and implementing mitigation techniques for additional vascular damage are all part of navigating vascular dementia.

Memory of Lewy Bodies:
Lewy bodies, aberrant protein deposits in the brain, are a hallmark of Lewy Body Dementia (LBD). It has characteristics in common with both Parkinson's and Alzheimer's diseases, which results in a distinct set of symptoms, such as visual hallucinations, changes in cognitive function, and movement difficulties. Managing LBD involves being aware of how it fluctuates, using specific strategies to deal with hallucinations, and taking into account how it affects both motor and cognitive performance.

Dementia Frontotemporal:
The frontal and temporal lobes of the brain are the main areas affected by frontotemporal dementia, which results in alterations in behavior, personality, and language. Compared to other varieties of dementia, this one frequently appears earlier in life.

Managing frontotemporal dementia entails tackling the behavioral and social issues it causes, comprehending how it affects connections with others, and investigating helpful techniques for both the affected person and their carers.

Combination Dementia:
A person with mixed dementia displays characteristics of multiple dementia types at the same time. Vascular dementia and Alzheimer's disease frequently coexist. Handling the distinct obstacles presented by every subtype of dementia, separating out the numerous contributing causes, and customizing interventions according to the intricate interaction of diseases are all part of managing mixed dementia.

Parkinson's illness Dementia: Parkinson's disease, a movement illness, has the potential to advance to dementia and cognitive deterioration. Along with cognitive impairment, people with Parkinson's disease dementia may also have movement symptoms. Parkinson's disease dementia necessitates a comprehensive strategy that takes into account the effects on quality of life and day-to-day functioning, addressing both motor and cognitive elements.

Disease of Huntington's
The inherited disorder known as Huntington's disease is marked by gradual motor dysfunction, cognitive impairment, and psychological problems. Managing motor symptoms, genetic counseling, and the

psychosocial effects on patients and their families are all important aspects of managing Huntington's disease.

Creutzfeldt-Jakob illness: A uncommon and quickly developing prion illness affecting the brain is called Kreutzfeldt-Jakob disease. It causes a reduction in both motor and cognitive function. Handling the special difficulties brought on by its quick progression and providing supportive care are essential to managing this difficult diagnosis.

Wernicke-Korsakoff Syndrome: This condition, which is typified by memory loss, confusion, and neurological symptoms, is frequently linked to long-term alcohol usage. Navigating this syndrome entails addressing nutritional inadequacies, controlling cognitive symptoms, and researching strategies to promote general health.

In summary, navigating the many forms of dementia necessitates a sophisticated comprehension of the varied terrain these subtypes cover. Every kind offers unique difficulties, diagnostic implications, and ramifications for people and their families. A comprehensive and compassionate approach to treatment and support is fostered by the journey's customized approaches, which address the distinctive manifestations of each subtype. The taxonomy of dementia kinds continues to change as research and knowledge expand, providing hope for more accurate diagnosis, focused interventions, and enhanced quality of life for those living with these complicated disorders.

CHAPTER SIX

Treatment Strategies for Cognitive Decline

The complex problem of cognitive decline, which affects people of all ages and neurological disorders, calls for a careful examination of possible interventions. This thorough analysis explores the complex field of interventions, tying together pharmacological strategies, dietary supplements, behavioral therapies, cognitive rehabilitation, social engagement, mindfulness exercises, sleep hygiene, and caregiver support. The main objective is to promote cognitive well-being by addressing the various factors that lead to cognitive deterioration as we make our way over this vast terrain.

Medical Interventions:
Medication intended to control neurotransmitter activity and lessen cognitive symptoms is the foundation of the pharmacological arm of managing cognitive decline. Memantine controls glutamate activity, and cholinesterase inhibitors like donepezil and rivastigmine work to raise acetylcholine levels. These drugs provide symptomatic relief and may reduce the progression of illnesses such as Alzheimer's disease, even if they are not curative. The

ever-evolving field of pharmaceutical research keeps presenting fresh opportunities for focused therapies.

Changes to Lifestyle:
Accepting changes to one's lifestyle becomes an essential cornerstone in the quest for cognitive wellness. Frequent exercise has been shown to improve cardiovascular health, support neuroplasticity, increase blood flow to the brain, and slow down the aging process. Essential nutrition for brain health comes from a heart-healthy diet high in nutrient-dense foods, omega-3 fatty acids, and antioxidants. Lifestyle changes include puzzles, acquiring new skills, social connections, and other mental stimulation to maintain cognitive resilience in the face of decline.

Rehabilitation of the Brain:
Specialized treatments aimed at improving particular cognitive capacities prioritize cognitive rehabilitation. These organized therapies target areas like memory, attention, and problem-solving and are tailored to each person's strengths and weaknesses. Beyond just treating symptoms, cognitive rehabilitation aims to maximize day-to-day functioning through the development of compensatory and adaptive mechanisms that are specific to each person's individual cognitive profile.

Behavioral Strategies:

Behavioral therapies resonate with the emotional and behavioral aspects of cognitive decline. Fostering emotional well-being, controlling stress, and treating mood disorders all help to create a supportive atmosphere. Behavioral techniques explore the complex relationship between emotional states and cognitive function, providing a comprehensive approach to controlling cognitive decline. These strategies include cognitive-behavioral therapy, counseling, and psychosocial interventions.

Support for Nutrition:
Support from nutrition appears to be essential for maintaining cognitive health. Dietary patterns like the Mediterranean diet highlight the benefits of antioxidant-rich foods, omega-3 fatty acids, and minerals that fuel the brain for improved cognitive function. Supplementation under the supervision of medical professionals becomes a targeted technique to address specific demands and maintain general cognitive health in cases where nutritional inadequacies lead to cognitive decline.

Interaction with Society:
Keeping up social ties is important for cognitive health and goes beyond being just a social grace. A sense of purpose, emotional support, and cognitive stimulation are all provided by social involvement. Engaging in social events, organizations, and community activities creates a network of support that lowers feelings of loneliness and improves cognitive well-being by

fostering meaningful connections and shared experiences.

Reduction of Stress and Mindfulness:
Meditation and stress-reduction methods are examples of mindfulness activities that provide a reflective path toward cognitive well-being. These techniques encourage calmness, lower stress levels, and might have a favorable impact on cognitive performance. The complex web of managing cognitive decline incorporates mindfulness-based therapies, which recognize the relationship between mental and emotional wellness and cognitive function.

Hygiene of Sleep:
Getting enough good sleep is crucial for maintaining brain health and cognitive function, even though its importance is sometimes overlooked. Sleep problems, which are frequent with cognitive decline, can make symptoms worse and create a vicious cycle. A crucial tactic to support cognitive well-being is to establish appropriate sleep hygiene practices, which include keeping a regular sleep schedule, establishing a sleep-friendly atmosphere, and treating underlying sleep disorders.

Education and Support for Caregivers:
Considering that people with cognitive decline and their carers have a symbiotic relationship, caregiver education and support are essential components of the treatment paradigm. Support groups, educational

materials, and respite care services are beneficial to caregivers because they help them deal with the practical and emotional difficulties of providing care. A compassionate and knowledgeable caregiving environment is enhanced when caregivers get education and support, which improves the overall quality of care given to patients experiencing cognitive impairment.

To sum up, a thorough investigation into cognitive decline therapy methods presents a mosaic of interrelated techniques. A comprehensive effort to promote cognitive well-being is represented by the integration of pharmaceutical interventions, dietary support, behavioral interventions, cognitive rehabilitation, social engagement, mindfulness practices, sleep hygiene, and caregiver support. The field of managing cognitive decline is constantly changing due to scientific advancements, clinical insights, and tailored interventions. These developments offer promise for better approaches, higher quality of life, and a shared commitment to fostering cognitive resilience throughout life.

CHAPTER SEVEN

Lifestyle Interventions and Dementia Prevention

Strengthening Mental Health

Lifestyle treatments are effective weapons in the fight against dementia because they enable people to actively participate in maintaining their cognitive health. In examining the complex relationship between lifestyle decisions and dementia risk, this paper highlights the interdependence of physical health, mental stimulation, social interaction, and general well-being. As we explore the nuances of lifestyle interventions, the story takes shape as an active quest to develop routines that foster cognitive resilience.

Activities Physically:
Frequent exercise turns out to be a key component in preventing dementia. Exercise not only improves cardiovascular health but also increases cerebral blood flow, supports neuroplasticity, and stimulates the production of new neurons. Exercises like swimming, brisk walking, and aerobics not only improve physical fitness but also work as a powerful preventative measure against cognitive deterioration.

Nutritious Food:
One cannot stress the importance of maintaining a good diet in preventing dementia. Changing to a diet high in omega-3 fatty acids, antioxidants, and other necessary nutrients promotes brain function. The Mediterranean diet, which is high in whole grains, lean meats, fruits, and vegetables, has drawn interest because it may lower the risk of cognitive decline. A healthy brain becomes an enduring barrier against the effects of aging and neurodegenerative diseases.

Cognitive Stimulation: Engaging in cognitive activities and lifetime learning can serve as a proactive means of preventing dementia. Completing puzzles, reading, picking up new skills, or following hobbies are examples of activities that excite the brain, promote neuroplasticity, and increase cognitive reserve. By serving as a buffer, this cognitive reserve enables people to more resiliently face the effects of age-related changes or neurological disorders.

Interaction with Society:
Keeping up social ties is a powerful tool in the fight against dementia. A sense of purpose, emotional support, and cognitive stimulation are all provided by social involvement. Engaging in social events, becoming a member of organizations, volunteering, or cultivating connections within the community all contribute to a thriving social network that acts as a buffer against the loneliness frequently linked to cognitive impairment.

Relaxed Sleep:
One of the most important components of dementia prevention is the healing power of good sleep. The general health of the brain is influenced by developing appropriate sleep hygiene habits, keeping a regular sleep schedule, and setting up a comfortable sleeping environment. Sufficient sleep promotes cellular repair, emotional control, and memory consolidation, strengthening the brain's resistance to the cumulative impact of stressors.

Handling Stress:
Stress management is an essential lifestyle intervention since long-term stress is associated with a danger to cognitive health. Techniques for mindfulness, meditation, yoga, and relaxation turn into useful instruments in lessening the negative effects of stress on the brain. People strengthen their cognitive well-being and help prevent dementia by learning to be resilient in the face of adversity.

Reducing Tobacco and Alcohol Consumption:
Preventing dementia requires addressing modifiable risk factors, such as abstaining from tobacco and alcohol usage. Smoking and excessive alcohol consumption are linked to a higher risk of cognitive deterioration. A lifestyle that places a high value on moderation and giving up bad habits improves general health and strengthens cognitive resilience.

Regular Health Check-ups: Proactive management of chronic illnesses along with regular health check-ups help prevent dementia. Maintaining cardiovascular health and lowering the risk of vascular-related cognitive decline are achieved by treating illnesses such as hypertension, diabetes, and high cholesterol with medication, lifestyle modifications, and following physician recommendations.

To sum up, lifestyle modifications aimed at preventing dementia are a proactive and powerful strategy for maintaining cognitive health. A comprehensive approach combines cognitive stimulation, social interaction, physical activity, healthy eating, stress reduction, and conscientious health habits. Adopting these lifestyle treatments becomes a transforming act of self-care as people traverse the aging process; it fosters cognitive resilience and promotes a lively and fulfilling quality of life. The story of dementia prevention is told via the dynamic interaction of decision-making, personal development, and a dedication to fostering the mental toughness that enriches the quality of our common human experience.

CHAPTER EIGHT

Supporting Individuals and Caregivers

A Caring Structure

Health issues, especially those related to cognitive decline, are not personal experiences; rather, they are a shared story between patients and the people who support them. The compassionate framework for assisting those with health concerns as well as the caregivers who are essential in their life is examined in this note. This framework seeks to enhance an atmosphere of comprehension, compassion, and comprehensive treatment by attending to the various requirements, psychological intricacies, and pragmatic obstacles.

Personal Assistance:

1. Building Self-Sufficiency: - It is critical to acknowledge and honor the autonomy of those who are dealing with health issues. Enhancing a person's feeling of agency and dignity involves giving them the freedom to voice their preferences, make decisions about their care, and actively participate in conversations about their well-being.

2. Customized Care Programs: Since each person's journey is different, care plans should be customized to meet their individual requirements. This calls for a cooperative strategy that takes into account the patient's aspirations for their quality of life as well as their medical needs, emotional health, and personal preferences.

3. Clear Communication: - Opening up lines of communication that are transparent and unobstructed is essential. A sense of control and comprehension is enhanced by having regular conversations with healthcare practitioners, including people in decision-making processes, and giving them clear information about their health.

4. Well-Being Holistic: A person's mental, emotional, and social needs must be taken into account when managing their holistic well-being in addition to their medical needs. A happy and fulfilled existence is enhanced by joyful pursuits, chances for social connection, and intellectual stimulation.

Help for Caregivers:

1. Emotional Sturdiness: Caregivers frequently traverse difficult emotional terrain. Recognizing their emotions, lending a sympathetic ear, and creating a secure environment in which they may share their worries, disappointments, and pleasures are all parts

of providing emotional support. Empathy and comprehension foster emotional resilience.

2. Education and Resources: - It is essential to provide caregivers with knowledge and tools. This includes factual information regarding the illness, a list of the support resources that are available, and helpful advice on chores related to providing care. Caretakers are more equipped to carry out their tasks when they are knowledgeable.

3. Respite Care: - In order to take care of their own wellbeing, caregivers need brief breaks. Caretakers can have a break and recharge with the help of respite care services, which can be provided by family members, the community, or professional caregivers.

4. Community and Peer Support: - Creating a network of support, such as peer networks and community groups, helps caregivers connect with others going through comparable struggles. Mutual understanding, guidance, and shared experiences help caregivers feel less alone and more like a part of the community.

5. Training and Skill Development: - Giving caregivers access to chances for skill development and training boosts their self-assurance and competency in providing care. This could involve instructions on how to manage particular illnesses, follow medical procedures, or even practice effective communication.

Cooperative Method:

1. Multidisciplinary Groups: - A comprehensive support system is ensured by a collaborative and interdisciplinary approach combining social workers, counselors, healthcare experts, and support groups. The combined knowledge covers a wide range of care demands, from physical health to mental health.

2. Personalized Care Programs: - Individualized care plans take into account the requirements of the caregiver as well as the individual since they acknowledge that every caring journey is different. An adaptable care plan that can be modified to accommodate changing needs makes the support system more efficient and responsive.

3. Continuous Communication: - It's critical to keep lines of communication open between patients, caregivers, and healthcare professionals. The care team builds trust and teamwork through regular updates, check-ins, and flexibility in meeting changing needs.

To sum up, providing care for both patients and carers necessitates a kind and comprehensive framework that takes into account the many facets of health issues. We support a collaborative approach, recognize the emotional complexity of caregivers, and empower individuals to create a caring atmosphere that is marked by empathy, understanding, and a dedication to improving the general well-being of persons navigating health journeys.

CHAPTER NINE

Advances in Dementia Research

Providing Light on the Way to Hope and Understanding

Unprecedented advancements in dementia research are shedding light on the complicated processes underlying this disorder, and the field is currently entering a revolutionary period. This paper examines the state-of-the-art in dementia research, highlighting innovations, new technologies, and cooperative efforts that could advance our knowledge and provide hope for creative interventions.

Genetic Discoveries: New findings about the inherited components of dementia have been made possible by advances in genetic research. The discovery of particular genetic abnormalities linked to Alzheimer's disease and other dementias in families has created opportunities for early detection, customized risk assessments, and focused treatment approaches. Genetic discoveries help to understand the underlying causes of dementia and can inform customized therapies.

Exploration of Biomarkers:

The search for trustworthy biomarkers has accelerated since they may provide instruments for monitoring the course of a disease and making early diagnoses. Advanced imaging methods including positron emission tomography (PET) and indicators of the cerebrospinal fluid, blood, and other tissues help to clarify the biochemical and anatomical alterations linked to various forms of dementia. Early detection made possible by these biomarkers opens the door to prompt interventions and individualized treatment plans.

Techniques for Neuroimaging:
Technological advancements in neuroimaging have completely changed our capacity to see the composition and operation of the brain. Advanced diffusion tensor imaging, functional magnetic resonance imaging (fMRI), and high-resolution MRI offer previously unattainable insights into the complex networks and connection patterns found in the brain. These imaging tools provide a visible road map for focused therapies and advance our knowledge of how neurodegenerative processes develop.

Approaches in Precision Medicine:
Precision medicine is bringing dementia research into the modern era by customizing interventions based on patient differences in genetics, biomarkers, and therapy response. Personalized methods take into account each person's distinct genetic composition, molecular profile, and lifestyle choices, opening the

door to more focused and successful treatment plans. By maximizing therapeutic results and reducing adverse effects, precision medicine has the potential to completely transform the way dementia is treated.

Medicine Research and Clinical Trials:
There is a current wave of drug research projects in the pharmaceutical industry that focus on several facets of dementia pathophysiology. Novel chemicals with the goals of altering the course of a disease, reducing symptoms, and targeting certain biological targets are being investigated in ongoing clinical trials. A strong pipeline of possible therapeutics is a result of cooperation between academic institutions, business, and regulatory agencies; this gives hope for successful disease-modifying drugs.

Machine learning and artificial intelligence:
In the field of dementia research, machine learning and artificial intelligence (AI) have become formidable companions. With previously unheard-of accuracy, these systems analyze enormous databases, spot trends, and forecast disease trajectories. Algorithms powered by AI are helpful in risk assessment, early diagnosis, and spotting tiny cognitive alterations that might be signs of something more serious before symptoms manifest. AI-enabled dementia research improves diagnosis accuracy and speeds up the identification of new treatment targets.

Lifestyle Interventions and Risk Reduction: There has been a surge in interest in the relationship between lifestyle factors and dementia risk. Research on the protective effects of food, social interaction, cognitive stimulation, and physical activity against cognitive decline provides useful information for prophylactic approaches. Comprehending the impact of lifestyle alterations on brain health serves as a basis for both customized therapies and public health campaigns.

Global Partnerships and Information Exchange:
Through global initiatives and data-sharing networks, the collaborative spirit in dementia research has blossomed. Scholars from throughout the globe collaborate to share data, pool resources, and take on the global crisis of dementia. Cohort studies with a large sample size, like the Alzheimer's Disease Neuroimaging Initiative (ADNI), encourage teamwork, which speeds up research and strengthens the community's resolve to advance dementia studies.

To sum up, the progress made in the field of dementia research is encouraging since it sheds light on the complex processes that underlie cognitive decline. The combined efforts of the scientific community are breaking new ground in a variety of fields, including precision medicine, advanced neuroimaging technology, genetic discoveries, and biomarker research. These discoveries not only broaden our understanding of dementia but also give hope for a time when individualized care plans and creative interventions will revolutionize the field of dementia research.

CHAPTER TEN

Cognitive Rehabilitation Techniques

Fostering Neuroplasticity and Self-Sufficiency
The goal of cognitive rehabilitation procedures is to improve cognitive performance, lessen impairments, and foster functional independence. They are a dynamic and ever-evolving set of interventions. These methods, which are based on the idea of neuroplasticity—the brain's capacity for adaptation and reorganization—offer specialized approaches to deal with various cognitive difficulties. In order to empower people with cognitive impairments, this note examines the fundamental ideas and many methodologies in the field of cognitive rehabilitation.

Cognitive Rehabilitation Principles:

1. Neurodiversity: - The fundamental idea of cognitive rehabilitation is called neuroplasticity, which refers to the brain's amazing ability to change and rearrange itself in response to events and difficulties. By utilizing this innate plasticity, cognitive rehabilitation encourages beneficial alterations in brain networks that support healing and adaptability.

2. Individualization: - It is essential to acknowledge that every person has a distinct cognitive profile. Since cognitive impairments vary widely among conditions and people, cognitive rehabilitation treatments are customized to address particular cognitive strengths and problems.

3. Aim-focused Method: - Cognitive rehabilitation is based on a goal-oriented approach. Collaboratively creating attainable and significant goals with others promotes motivation and involvement. Objectives may cover a range of cognitive areas, including problem-solving, executive function, memory, and attention.

Important Methods for Cognitive Rehabilitation:

1. Memory Techniques: Memory impairments are a widespread problem, and compensatory measures are the main focus of rehabilitation approaches. These include memory aides, spaced retrieval strategies, and mnemonic devices to enhance information encoding, storage, and retrieval.

2. Attentive Education: - Training methods focus on improving divided, sustained, and selective attention since attention is an important cognitive function. Attentional improvements are facilitated by tasks that involve concentrated attention exercises, attention-shifting drills, and dual-task activities.

3. Executive Function Training: - Activities aimed at improving planning, organizing, problem-solving, and decision-making are part of executive function rehabilitation. Executive skill growth and improvement are supported by real-world simulations, structured exercises, and cognitive-behavioral techniques.

4. Cognitive activities and Games: - Games and activities that need active cognitive function offer a stimulating setting for recovery. Overall cognitive well-being is enhanced by engaging in activities that test logical thinking, spatial awareness, and reasoning.

5. Interventions Based on Technology: - Virtual reality applications and apps for cognitive training have been made possible by technological advancements. These treatments give cognitive exercise platforms that are interactive and adaptable, adding more choices for rehabilitation in a variety of contexts.

6. Reminiscence therapy and reality orientation: - Reminiscence therapy and reality orientation are helpful strategies for those with cognitive deterioration. Reminiscence therapy uses recollections of the past to promote emotional and cognitive well-being, whereas reality orientation uses knowledge about time, place, and people to improve orientation.

7. Social Cognitive Training: - The goals of social cognitive training are to enhance social

communication, emotion recognition, and interpersonal skills. Improved social interactions and adaptive behaviors can be attributed to role-playing, group activities, and social skills training.

8. Multimodal Approaches: - A multimodal approach acknowledges the interdependence of cognitive functions by combining different cognitive rehabilitation strategies. For example, the synergistic effect on general cognitive capacities is enhanced when memory exercises are combined with attention training.

Applicability in Various Situations:

1. Stroke Rehabilitation: - Cognitive rehabilitation, which addresses cognitive deficiencies resulting from vascular injury, is essential to stroke recovery. Strategies concentrate on regaining cognitive function and adjusting to the difficulties brought on by the brain damage caused by the stroke.

2. Brain Injury (Traumatic Brain Injury): People who have had traumatic brain injuries frequently have a variety of cognitive deficits. Memory, attention, and executive function difficulties are addressed by cognitive rehabilitation approaches that are customized to the individual cognitive domains compromised.

3. Neurodegenerative Conditions: - Cognitive rehabilitation attempts to maximize residual abilities, postpone further decline, and improve quality of life through adaptive strategies and cognitive exercises in neurodegenerative conditions like Alzheimer's disease, where progressive cognitive decline is evident.

4. Psychiatric Disorders: - Cognitive rehabilitation strategies may be helpful for psychiatric disorders that involve cognitive elements, such as bipolar disorder or schizophrenia. Improving functional results and day-to-day living abilities is facilitated by addressing cognitive deficiencies linked to these diseases.

To sum up, cognitive rehabilitation methods represent a flexible and customized strategy for promoting neuroplasticity and functional independence. These methods, which have their roots in neuroplastic adaptation theory, give people who are struggling with cognitive issues in a variety of settings hope and a sense of empowerment. Enhancing cognitive well-being and improving overall quality of life through tailored interventions, meaningful goal-setting, and recognition of personal strengths make cognitive rehabilitation a transforming process.

CHAPTER ELEVEN

Ethical Considerations in Dementia Care

How to Make Compassionate Decisions

The care of those with dementia is a challenging ethical terrain that must be carefully navigated while putting the needs of those experiencing cognitive decline, their autonomy, and their dignity first. This paper delves into the complex ethical issues surrounding dementia care, highlighting the significance of person-centered approaches, respectful decision-making, and maintaining dignity throughout the caregiving process.

Valuing Individuality:

1. Preventive Healthcare Planning: - Encouraging advance care planning conversations is the first step toward respecting autonomy. People's desires are taken into consideration and respected when they are encouraged to communicate their preferences on treatment alternatives, end-of-life care, and future medical decisions.

2. Informed Consent: - A fundamental component of moral dementia care is informed consent. To ensure

that people retain agency in topics affecting their lives, caregivers and healthcare professionals must ensure that information is communicated effectively, involve people in decision-making as much as possible, and get consent for medical interventions.

Maintaining Dignity:

1. Person-Centered Care: – This approach puts the patient at the center of the decision-making process. Preserving dignity and promoting a sense of identity in individuals with dementia can be achieved through customization of care plans, activities, and communication styles based on their choices, values, and life history.

2. Respecting Cultural and Spiritual Beliefs: - It's important to acknowledge and honor people's cultural and spiritual beliefs. In addition to recognizing the diversity of viewpoints, ethical dementia care makes ensuring that the cultural and spiritual values of the people it is providing are respected.

Keeping Safety and Autonomy in Check:

1. Community and Home-Based Care: - It's important to strike a balance between the need for autonomy and safety, especially in home and community-based care settings. Making ethical decisions entails evaluating the dangers, putting safety measures in

place, and enabling people to stay in familiar surroundings while still feeling reasonably safe.

2. Wandering and Restraint Use: - When discussing wandering habits and the application of restrictions, ethical issues come up. Prioritizing the exploration of alternative techniques, such as tailored interventions or environmental alterations, over the consideration of restrictive measures is crucial in striking a balance between the promotion of safety and the respect for autonomy.

Dedications at the End of Life:

1. Palliative and Hospice Care: - When appropriate, a careful transition to palliative and hospice care is part of ethical decision-making at the end of life. It is crucial to make sure that the emphasis moves from curative efforts to comfort, dignity, and quality of life in order to promote a humane and respectable dying process.

2. Withholding or Withdrawing Treatment: - Careful consideration of the patient's values, quality of life, and preferences is necessary when making decisions about withholding or withdrawing treatment. Discussions regarding the appropriateness of interventions are guided by ethical frameworks, which acknowledge that forceful medical measures are frequently subordinated in favor of comfort and dignity.

Informed Decision-Making and Communication:

1. Clear Communication: - Clear and sympathetic contacts with people who have dementia and their families are a crucial component of ethical communication. Healthcare providers and carers ought to address concerns, facilitate joint decision-making, and communicate information in an intelligible manner.

2. Advocacy and Proxy Decision-Making: - Situations when people might not be able to make decisions on their own are covered by ethical issues. Ethical standards in dementia care are upheld by designating trusted advocates, having prior discussions on proxy decision-making, and making sure that decisions are in line with the patient's values.

Reducing Shame and Encouraging Inclusion:

1. De-Stigmatizing: - The goal of ethical dementia care is to lessen the stigma attached to cognitive decline. Encouraging awareness, education, and community involvement creates an atmosphere where people with dementia are treated with respect, understanding, and dignity.

2. Social and Community participation: - Encouraging social and community participation is beneficial to the wellbeing of people living with dementia. The

significance of developing inclusive environments that value the person beyond their diagnosis, encouraging social interactions, and lessening isolation is emphasized by ethical considerations.

To sum up, ethical issues surrounding dementia care highlight how important it is to maintain dignity, strike a balance between safety and autonomy, and protect the rights of those who are experiencing cognitive loss. Ethical caregiving becomes a compass in the complex world of dementia care by adopting person-centered approaches, honoring cultural and spiritual beliefs, and making compassionate judgments about end-of-life care. Ethical standards become essential components of holistic and compassionate assistance for persons and their families during the dementia journey through deliberate decision-making and advocacy.

CONCLUSION

Empowering Lives Through Understanding

Understanding becomes the cornerstone in the intricate web of dementia care, connecting ethical considerations, knowledge, and compassion. The experience of cognitive decline is complex and affects people's lives as well as that of their carers and communities. As we come to the end of this investigation, the story becomes clear as evidence of the transforming potential of knowledge in enhancing the lives of those impacted by dementia.

Empathetic Perception:
Effective dementia care is centered on compassion. A compassionate atmosphere is fostered by an understanding of the emotional complexities, problems, and triumphs faced by persons and their caregivers. By recognizing the humanity in the diagnosis, it promotes a bond and a sense of humanity that goes beyond cognitive deterioration.

Awareness as a Facilitator:
Empowerment is triggered by knowledge. A solid understanding of dementia gives communities, healthcare providers, and caregivers the ability to manage the challenges of cognitive decline. This

includes understanding the nuances of cognitive rehabilitation methods as well as the latest developments in dementia research. A shared dedication to lifelong learning leads to well-informed choices, tailored interventions, and creative solutions.

Basics of Ethics:
The direction of dementia care is determined by ethical considerations, which act as guiding principles and provide integrity and respect. Maintaining dignity in all decisions, striking a balance between autonomy and safety, and acknowledging the cultural and spiritual aspects of care are the ethical cornerstones that support a person-centered and compassionate approach.

Building Up Lives:
Empowerment emerges as the main objective. Person-centered care, tailored interventions, and a dedication to lowering stigma provide opportunities for fulfillment and enrichment for those impacted by dementia. Empowerment is a journey, not a destination, that honors the individuality, resiliency, and qualities of every person dealing with cognitive decline.

Comprehensive Neighborhoods:
Understanding encompasses communities in addition to individual care. An environment that is supportive is enhanced by inclusive settings that lessen stigma, encourage social interaction, and raise awareness.

Building diverse and inclusive societies and appreciating the value and contributions of people regardless of their cognitive health state are essential to empowering lives via understanding.

Complete Wellness:
Promoting comprehensive well-being and seeking understanding are mutually exclusive in the context of dementia care. The concept of well-being extends beyond the clinical setting and includes strategies such as lifestyle treatments that support both physical and mental health and cognitive rehabilitation procedures that foster neuroplasticity. It embraces the diversity of life and the interrelated aspects of mental, emotional, social, and spiritual well-being.

A Joint Obligation:
Caregivers, medical professionals, researchers, and communities all have a shared commitment to empowering lives through understanding. It recognizes that everyone must do their part to make the world a place where people who are experiencing cognitive decline are respected, understood, and seen. This dedication is evident in the cooperative initiatives to progress medical knowledge, improve healthcare procedures, and create inclusive communities.

Thinking back on the trip through the domains of cognitive decline, understanding that is compassionate comes to light as a ray of hope. It is the power that turns obstacles into chances, hardships into fortitude, and intimate encounters into a fabric of our common humanity. By empowering lives with understanding, we improve the quality of life for everyone impacted by the complicated journey of cognitive decline by navigating the challenges of dementia and weaving a story of compassion, knowledge, and moral care.

www.ingramcontent.com/pod-product-compliance
Lightning Source LLC
Chambersburg PA
CBHW050850260726
48660CB00006B/2553